Health Benefits Of Intermittent Fasting

The understanding of Intermittent Fasting and its health benefit to our body

Table of Contents

What is Intermittent Fasting (IF)?

The word "Intermittent" is defined as "occurring in irregular intervals." The word fasting is an act in which one refrains from a certain activity for a specific period of time. Simply put Intermittent Fasting is refraining from food for a certain time period.

Intermittent Fasting (IF) has two components

- A fasting period: time interval in which you refrain from eating

- A feeding window: time interval in which you are allowed to eat.

What Intermittent Fasting (IF) is not?

- IF is not a magic bullet for weight loss, you will not lose 10lbs in one week. You may, however, make consistent loss such as 1pound per week.

- IF does not claim to be the best diet or the best approach to dieting for everyone. IF is a simplified diet method that works best for the busy individual.

- IF is not a necessity. IF, like every other diet is just a tool to help you lose weight. Think of it as another tool to add to your toolbox for fat-loss. There are plenty of other ways to lose weight.

Why should you fast?

Intermittent fasting has many benefits, here are a few.

- Lower blood pressure

- Lower oxidative stress

- Increased fat burning

- Increased metabolic rate during the fast

- Improved appetite control

- Improved blood sugar control

- Improved cardiovascular function

Who is this ebook for?

This manual is for those who

- Want to learn the basic of intermittent fasting

- Want a to improve their health

- Experience a consistent and manageable way to lose weight

Chapter 1

Understanding All About Intermittent Fasting

Intermittent Fasting (IF) refers to dietary eating patterns that involve not eating or severely restricting calories for a prolonged period of time. There are many different subgroups of intermittent fasting each with individual variation in the duration of the fast; some for hours, others for the day(s). This has become an extremely popular topic in the science community due to all of the potential benefits on fitness and health that are being discovered.

What is intermittent fasting?

The main reason for following a fasting diet (of which there are lots of versions) is to improve regulation of insulin levels by balancing times of feeding and fasting. Insulin is an anabolic hormone which promotes the storage of nutrients (including fat). When levels of insulin are high, like they are following a meal or snack*, we are not able to burn fat. Fasting for extended periods allows our insulin levels to drop, resulting in periods where we are able to use our body's fat stores as energy. Fasting can therefore be beneficial for weight loss and for preventing insulin resistance; which is a key component of many health conditions.

Intermittent fasting is a pattern of eating. It's a way of scheduling your meals so that you get the most out of them. Intermittent fasting doesn't change what you eat, it changes when you eat.

Why is it worthwhile to change when you're eating?

Well, most notably, it's a great way to get lean without going on a crazy diet or cutting your calories down to nothing. In fact, most of the time you'll try to keep your calories the same when you start intermittent fasting. (Most people eat bigger meals during a shorter time frame.) Additionally, intermittent fasting is a good way to keep muscle mass on while getting lean.

Perhaps most importantly, intermittent fasting is one of the simplest strategies we have for taking bad weight off while keeping good weight on because it requires very little behavior change. This is a very good thing because it means intermittent fasting falls into the category of "simple enough that you'll actually do it, but meaningful enough that it will actually make a difference."

How Does Intermittent Fasting Work?

To understand how intermittent fasting leads to fat loss we first need to understand the difference between the fed state and the fasted state.

Your body is in the fed state when it is digesting and absorbing food. Typically, the fed state starts when you begin eating and lasts for three to five hours as your body digests and absorbs the food you just ate. When you are in the fed state, it's very hard for your body to burn fat because your insulin levels are high.

After that timespan, your body goes into what is known as the post–absorptive state, which is just a fancy way of saying that your body isn't processing a meal. The post–absorptive state lasts until 8 to 12 hours after your last meal, which is when you enter the fasted state. It is much easier for you body to burn fat in the fasted state because your insulin levels are low.

When you're in the fasted state your body can burn fat that has been inaccessible during the fed state.

Because we don't enter the fasted state until 12 hours after our last meal, it's rare that our bodies are in this fat burning state. This is one of the reasons why many people who start intermittent fasting will lose fat without changing what they eat, how much they eat, or how often they exercise. Fasting puts your body in a fat burning state that you rarely make it to during a normal eating schedule.

Intermittent Fasting And Health: What Is The Evidence?

Fasting has been practiced for centuries for both spiritual and health reasons, but intermittent fasting has only recently become popular, with a growing body of research indicating that there may be health benefits – to not only what we eat, but when we eat.

Intermittent fasting involves a regimen of eating for a specified time, and then abstaining from food altogether for another specified time period.

Intermittent fasting can be carried out as part of a daily routine, e.g., eating between the hours of 8 am to 6pm, and then abstaining from food between the hours of 6pm and 8am the next day. Length of time without food may vary from 12 to 18 hours each day, depending on individuals' state of health, goals, and preference.

Alternatively, intermittent fasting can involves eating every other day while fasting or greatly lowering food intake in between those days.

Research findings in animals, and to a more limited extent in humans, are providing evidence that intermittent fasting may improve risk markers for chronic disease, such as lowered cholesterol, reduced insulin resistance, and decreased blood pressure, as well as facilitate needed weight loss. There are also indications that fasting, including intermittent fasting, may improve mental function and decrease symptoms of depression.

Additionally, small trials are showing promise for the possible benefits of intermittent fasting or fasting mimicking diets in improving outcomes and lowering side effects in cancer patients using chemotherapy protocols.

Exciting research is also exploring the possible health benefits on intermittent fasting for enhancing longevity.

An important aspect of intermittent fasting is the ☐uality of one's diet, in terms of nutrient balance and nutrient density.

A number of excellent books and articles describe how to implement intermittent fasting, and report on the evidence backing up the benefits of this approach. In the column to the right, you will find a few publications you may wish to explore as you investigate intermittent fasting for yourself or your patients.

Types Of Intermittent Fasting

Intermittent fasting comes in various forms and each may have a specific set of uni□ue benefits. Each form of intermittent fasting has variations in the fasting-to-eating ratio. The benefits and effectiveness of these different protocols may differ on an individual basis and it is important to determine which one is best for you. Factors that may influence which one to choose includes health goals, daily schedule/routine, and current health status. The most common types of IF are alternate day fasting, time-restricted feeding, and modified fasting.

1. Alternate Day Fasting:

This approach involves alternating days of absolutely no calories (from food or beverage) with days of free feeding and eating whatever you want.

2. Modified Fasting - 5:2 Diet

Modified fasting is a protocol with programmed fasting days, but the fasting days do allow for some food intake.

3. Time-Restricted Feeding:

If you know anyone that has said they are doing intermittent fasting, odds are it is in the form of time-restricted feeding. This is a type of intermittent fasting that is used daily and it involves only consuming calories during a small portion of the day and fasting for the remainder.

Chapter 3

The Health Benefits of Intermittent Fasting

Unlike fad diets, fasting is not expensive, inconvenient, time consuming, complex or difficult. Intermittent fasting is accessible to everyone, all the time.

Research on intermittent fasting is in it's infancy but it still has huge potential for weight loss and the treatment of some chronic disease.

To recap, here are the possible health benefits of intermittent fasting:

Shown in Human Studies:

1. Weight loss

2. Improve blood lipid markers like cholesterol

3. Reduce inflammation

4. Reduced stress and improved self confidence

5. Improved mood

Shown in Animal Studies:

1. Decreased Body Fat

2. Decreased levels of the hunger hormone leptin

3. Improve insulin levels

4. Protect against obesity, fatty liver disease, and inflammation

5. Longevity

Health Benefits

Many studies have been done on intermittent fasting, in both animals and humans.

These studies have shown that it can have powerful benefits for weight control and the health of your body and brain. It may even help you live longer.

Here are the main health benefits of intermittent fasting:

- Weight loss: As mentioned above, intermittent fasting can help you lose weight and belly fat, without having to consciously restrict calories.

- Insulin resistance: Intermittent fasting can reduce insulin resistance, lowering blood sugar by 3–6% and fasting insulin levels by 20–31%, which should protect against type 2 diabetes.

- Inflammation: Some studies show reductions in markers of inflammation, a key driver of many chronic diseases.

- Heart health: Intermittent fasting may reduce "bad" LDL cholesterol, blood triglycerides, inflammatory markers, blood sugar and insulin resistance — all risk factors for heart disease.

- Brain health: Intermittent fasting increases the brain hormone BDNF and may aid the growth of new nerve cells. It may also protect against Alzheimer's disease.

- Anti-aging: Intermittent fasting can extend lifespan in rats. Studies showed that fasted rats lived 36–83% longer.

- Cancer: Animal studies suggest that intermittent fasting may prevent cancer.

Fat Loss: Intermittent Fasting For Weight Loss

Intermittent fasting helps your body become better adapted to oxidizing fat for energy. Because of the decreased window of time for eating, insulin levels are lower, allowing adipocytes (fat cells) to release fatty acids.

The lower levels of glucose and glycogen encourage the body to use these fatty acids to generate energy for the body and brain rather than store the fatty acids in fat cells.

You use up fat instead of storing it and soon burn what you've already stored.

Adherence is another important factor for IF as a tool for weight loss.

Studies confirm that people regain their previous weight or more, several years after a diet.

Why? They fail to adhere to their diets. That's not surprising, since most diets make long term adherence nearly impossible.

Intermittent fasting is comparably effortless to sustain, reducing calorie intake, inducing ketosis,

lipolysis, autophagy and other positive bodily responses that work together toward weight loss.

Intermittent Fasting For Weight Loss Tips

Intermittent fasting is without a doubt one of the fastest and most efficient ways to lose body-fat and do better. But how do you go about it? Here are 5 tips to help you get started on an effective intermittent fasting diet.

Don't make your fast too long or too short

An ideal fast length for weight-loss and health benefits is between 16 and 24 hours depending on age, experience and exact goals. Any less than this won't really give you the results you want (remember you are already fasting for 10-12 hours overnight) and any longer than this is simply unnecessary and can be harder to adapt to.

Increase your water intake when fasting

Intermittent fasting will also help to cleanse your system and let your body work more efficiently. In order to help this process, you should increase your water intake. The best way to do this is have a glass/bottle of water with you at all times so that you can sip regularly.

Break your fast with a healthy meal

The first thing you eat after a fat should be a healthy meal. Apart from the obvious benefits of eating healthy food, this also leaves less space for eating junk. Given that you might only have 8 hours to eat your daily food, filling up on the good stuff first is always a good option.

Time your food around your workouts

It goers without saying that working out should be part of any healthy eating plan. The centre piece of your training efforts should be weight-training or bodyweight training. Try to eat most of your food in the period immediately after your workout. In this way your body will be more likely to use these calories to rebuild and repair rather than be stocked as fat.

Don't sweat the details

One of the real benefits of intermittent fasting is that it is not necessary to count calories or grams of macronutrients. This can be a pain and makes diets difficult to stick to. Follow principles and the details will take care of themselves.

Intermittent Fasting for Disease Prevention

Recent studies emerge to support the use of intermittent fasting as a means of lowering blood glucose in diabetics and leading to overall improved health outcomes.

In particular, one study published in the World Journal of Diabetes found that subjects with type 2 diabetes mellitus implementing short-term daily IF significantly reduced body weight, fasting glucose and improved post-meal glucose variability.

IF has been shown to:

- o   Improve markers of stress resistance

- Lower inflammation and blood pressure

- Improve glucose circulation and lipid levels, leading to a lower risk for cardiovascular disease, neurological disorders (such as Alzheimer's and Parkinson's) and cancer

Intermittent Fasting for Anti-Aging

Aging is Western society's public enemy #1, so how would you feel if you stumbled across the secret key to anti-aging?

Well, you just did.

The anti-aging capabilities of IF are coming to light as more studies show that it has a profound ability to decrease blood pressure, reduce oxidative damage, improve insulin sensitivity and glucose uptake, and decrease fat mass - all factors that contribute to enhancing health and longevity.

Fasting is one of the biological stressors that triggers autophagy - a process where your body clears out dead or underperforming cells and regenerates and recycles damaged proteins.

Autophagy is extremely important and a natural process that plays a significant role in preventing diseases such as cancer, neurodegeneration, diabetes, cardiomyopathy, autoimmune diseases, liver disease and much more.

Many of the benefits of fasting are due to this essential, physiological processes. Intermittent Fasting for Therapeutic Benefits

Physical

Beyond its application for diabetes management, IF is also proven to be as effective as approved drugs for reducing seizures and seizure-related brain damage and for healing rheumatoid arthritis.

Additionally, research is beginning to emerge showing positive effects of alternate day fasting on reducing the toxic effects of chemotherapy and decreasing morbidity rates associated with cancer.

Spiritual

Fasting is a common spiritual cleansing practice that remains an integral part of nearly all religions around the world. It's interesting to think that all of these religions are independent and uni☐ue yet they all share the use of fasting to heal and promote wellness.

Some might argue that fasting is usually a practice of penance. That's true, yes, but penance is a means to an end. The end is forgiveness and peace, self-love, and well-being.

This observation in itself should represent the power of fasting!

Psychological

Fasting helps improve willpower through regularly exercising the self-control muscle. When you fast, you are consciously choosing not to eat and therefore taking control of your mind and training it just like you would train your muscles during an intense gym session.

As a result of this training, you learn how to control your own eating and you develop the power to control other aspects of your life as well.

One recent study found that women who practiced intermittent fasting had positive experiences associated with increased sense of achievement, pride, reward and control.

Willpower influences your sense of accomplishment and self-esteem through being able to exhibit self-control.

Self-control, as evidenced by many studies-- the most famous was the Marshmallow Test-- is one of the greatest predictors of happiness, success and □uality of life.

Breaking your fast also brings an incredible sense of gratitude for food, life and nourishing of your body.

Intermittent Fasting for Superior Mental Performance

Intermittent fasting improves cognitive function and helps boost brain power.

As mentioned earlier, IF induces neuronal autophagy which allows your brain cells to recycle and repair themselves for optimal function.

Studies have shown that interference of neuronal autophagy can lead to neurodegeneration causing your brain to function insufficiently and prevent you from performing at your full potential.

Intermittent fasting also increases a protein in the brain called brain-derived neurotrophic factor (BDNF).

This protein interacts with the parts of your brain that control learning, memory and cognitive function. Studies have shown that BDNF helps protect your brain cells and even stimulates the growth of new ones

IF also triggers ketogenesis, where your body turns to fat for energy, metabolizing fat into ketones. Ketones easily cross the blood-brain-barrier, feeding your brain and resulting in better mental acuity, energy and productivity.

Combined with a well formulated whole-foods diet, IF avoids the blood sugar spikes caused by a high carb diet, which leads to brain fog and low mood issues like depression.

Intermittent Fasting for Better Physical Fitness

Yup, intermittent fasting also holds benefits for your physical fitness, too. Including:

Better Metabolism

Intermittent fasting trains your mind and digestive system to get used to eating what you need for the day in a smaller window of time.

This promotes a healthy and proportional intake of food and calories. People who get used to fasting and also eat a ketogenic diet soon learn to only eat when hungry, not according to pre-established mealtimes or impulsive and mindless eating.

Popular belief that fasting negatively affects your metabolism is unfounded.

When done the right way, fasting actually helps improve metabolism and promote metabolic flexibility where your body has the machinery to use glucose or fats effectively for energy.

Better Wind and Endurance

Football players and other athletes build and maintain their "wind" by running and doing other cardio training exercises.

Known in fitness as VO2 max, this is the maximum amount of oxygen per minute, per kilogram of body weight that you use during intense exercise.

The more oxygen you can use at a time, the more work output you can perform. Your VO2 max level is a measure of fitness; elite endurance athletes have twice the VO2 capacity of untrained people.

Important Measurements While Fasting: Weight, Body Fat, Body Tape Measurement Weight

When you fast, you will lose water weight. This is because your body uses water to hold glycogen in your muscles and liver. When your glycogen stores deplete, there is less need for water to hold it.

That's why many people see large weight loss when they fast. After your fast, however, you'll gain that water weight back.

In fasting and in keto, you burn fat and may replace that with lean muscle. Muscle is heavier than fat. Unless you have a lot of fat to lose, take the scale numbers with a pinch of salt, and grab the tape measure instead.

Body tape measurement

After you lose all the water weight, you'll start seeing "modest" weight loss when you fast or go keto and you replace fat with muscle.

But body tape measurements are gratifying. They show you how far you've come from your previous waistline. When doing body tape measurements, consistency is key. Use the same tape measure, and lay it flat on the same spot as always. For your thighs, calves, biceps and arms, measure the dominant side (i.e., the right arm if you're right-handed).

Keep in mind that research is still in its early stages — Many of the studies were small, short-term or conducted in animals. Many questions have yet to be answered in higher quality human studies.

Intermittent fasting can have many benefits for your body and brain. It can cause weight loss and may reduce your risk of type 2 diabetes, heart disease, and cancer. It may also help you live longer.

Get Started with Intermittent Fasting

Intermittent fasting is a method with various formulas you can try to take advantage of the many proven benefits: weight loss, disease prevention/treatment, ketosis, better mental and physical performance and overall health and fitness.

How much and how fast results manifest may vary, and what you do eat during your eating windows should be optimal for your own unique body composition and daily caloric needs.

Be mindful and get a read of your tendencies toward food and what your body likes. If you fast for 24 hours to justify an unhealthy binge before or after-- that's a picture you don't want to be in.

If you would be so kind to please leave a review (even if negative) so I can know how to improve my writing also to know if you'd like more content such as this. Thank you for reading! Good luck with your intermittent fasting journey.

www.ingramcontent.com/pod-product-compliance
Lightning Source LLC
Chambersburg PA
CBHW051145250726
48655CB00007B/3246